I0555109

don't forget to breathe.

A book of poems and reflections created
to provide space for self-discovery.

Written by Ceyanna Dent

Notice: Neither the publisher nor the author is engaged in rendering professional advice or services to the individual reader. The ideas and suggestions in this book are not intended as a substitute for consulting a licensed professional. All matters regarding your health require medical supervision. Neither the publisher nor the author shall be liable or responsible for any loss or damage allegedly arising from any information or suggestion in this book.

Copyright © 2023 by Ceyanna Dent

All rights are reserved. No part of this publication may be reproduced, distributed, or transmitted in any form, or by any means, including photocopying, recording, or other electronic or mechanical methods, without the prior written permission of the publisher, except in the case of brief quotations, embedded in reviews and certain other non-commercial uses permitted by copyright law.

Copy Editor: Krista Jones High
Contributing Writers: EbaNee Bond, Vanessa Flowers

Library of Congress Control Number: 2023918709
ISBN:979-8-218-27501-3

Printed in the United States.

Published by White Paper Ink, LLC | Akron, Ohio
Website: www.whitepaperink.com
Email ceyanna@whitepaperink.com

DEDICATION

This work is dedicated to the love of my life, my mom -
Crystal Dent Conway.

contents

***

***

@dontforgettobreathereflections (Instagram)
#DFTBReflections

My Prayer

Dear Lord,

Please see my heart and the intention behind the queries I lay before you.

How do I move past chasing and envying the energy I seek, to possessing the energy I seek?
To appreciate the energy I bring to the world?
To attract the energy I need?

How do I move from a mind consumed with lack, to one filled with the limitless nature of your love?
To accept your love from others?
To love in a way more representative of you?
To become love?

How do I fully inhabit the purpose you have for my life?

Please see my heart.

Amen.

Introduction

These pages hold the hope of my earnest search for community - my community. To see and be seen. To remember and be reminded. To share and hope to inspire.

It is with certitude that I profess that all I have are questions, and with the prerequisite mustard seed faith that I believe my questions bring me closer to my center - God. Questions are my inhale. Words are my exhale. An intricate set of idiosyncrasies that ensure I don't forget to breathe, literally and metaphorically.

This book of poems is my offering to the plate of truth. These poems represent instances where I carved out time to be honest and open with myself. They are my armor against fear, shame, and all the lies that separate me from peace.

A prompt accompanies each poem to encourage you to reflect through writing - an invitation for your words to be as liberating for you as mine have been for me. The impact of these pages is almost solely based on how willing you are to surrender to the process of unfolding to yourself.

Every poem is an example of me unfolding to myself, while the reflections are my stream-of-consciousness writings to share honest insights and perspectives on the preceding poetry piece.

My hope is that you will use *don't forget to breathe.* to do the same for yourself. Prioritize you, one poem and reflection at a time. Give yourself space between each reflection to *see* yourself, cogitate, honor your challenges, and revere your growth.

May you receive *don't forget to breathe.* in the spirit in which it was created - love.

BLUE FLAMES

Put Fear's feet to the fire.
Make him tell the truth.
Make him open the door.

And

Tell the skeleton's human story.
Make him speak of the lives stolen to feed his ego.
Make him fill in all the holes from the bombs he's exploded in wars -
fought by dreamers, now deferred.

Make him return the treasures he covets.
Make him strip naked.

Where is his truth?

REFLECTION ONE

More times than I am happy to admit, I allow fear, guilt, shame, or anxiety to steal my moments for radical honesty, opportunity, and growth. Those are the interactions I ruminate over, even though they do not represent the lion's share of my life experiences. This poem recounts a time when I personified one of my "moment stealers" - fear, to take back some of the power I had given to it.

Get settled into a physical space where you feel safe. Reflect on a moment when you conquered your Goliath - e.g. negative thoughts - with courage.

don't forget to breathe.

STRANGER TO ME TOO

I wish I knew you better,
like I know my thoughts,
my hopes,
my dreams.

I wish you didn't make me feel so foreign,
with your stretchy skin
and short limbs.

I wish I noticed you,
like the trips I take through my mind,
when I imagine another place,
or another world.

I wish I cherished you,
like when I stumble
onto a worldly connection,
an epiphany, or a word.

I wish I loved you,
like the feeling of worth
when a message from "that person"
flashes across my screen.

I wish I knew you better,
like I know my thoughts,
my hopes,
my dreams.

REFLECTION TWO

Stranger to Me Too is a poem born out of the estranged relationship between me and my body. It has been a multi-decade battle, full of landmines, fun house mirrors, improper internalizations, judgments from suitors unsuitable for me, and more. Fortunately, the story of me and my relationship with my body is still being written, so there is hope - this is where I would like to focus.

"To cherish a desire with anticipation" is how Merriam-Webster's dictionary defines hope. A secondary definition defines hope as "trust". What in your life provides you with hope? In what areas would you like to have more hope?

don't forget to breathe.

MOTHER NATURE

Before she gave her the world,
she sat her beside the fire:

and let her skin warm,
and her brown eyes twinkle,
and her coos follow the crackles,
and her hands mimic the flames,
and her spirit rise like embers...

Before day conquered the night,
and the world was hers.

REFLECTION THREE

Thursday happens to be my favorite day of the week. What I love most is the idea that my weekend is still full of possibilities - adventure, new memories, a little excitement. Additionally, Thursdays hold a nostalgia from my childhood, of watching new episodes of series like *The Cosby Show, A Different World, Martin,* and *Living Single* with my family. Like this poem, Thursdays dually represent what is to come, along with the memories I hold near.

What is your "Thursday"? Spend some time exploring what you hold in high regard, as well as what you wait for, with great anticipation.

don't forget to breathe.

MORNING PROVOCATION

I love him across planes,
and in total disregard of time.

There is no space between him and I,
only the illusion of apartness.

We share every moment.

I decided to carry him in love, as love,
and separately, him I.
(for eternity)

It settles my heart,
and calms my spirit.

It heals my soul,
and provides all of me peace.

This love is everything.

A total sum of all things,
and present in each and every one.

We travel across planes,
and through time.

Love is him,
and *he* is everything.

REFLECTION FOUR

Sometimes, my thoughts race at night, which doubles as the top of the morning. They range from unresolved concerns from the previous day to angst over the uncontrollable. These thoughts rarely inspire me to write. But every now and then, the thoughts feel more like messages using me as a portal to enter the world. They fill me with a sense of duty, of joy for feeling useful. They reflect the joy that fills me when a Baha'i prayer is read or sung by a member of the SisterNet* community during one of our weekly meetings. It is a feeling that calls me to obedience, begs me to capture the thoughts for future reflection, and allows me to remember - spiritually, ancestrally.

Not considering your life responsibilities, what repeatedly moves you/calls you to action?

*SisterNet: A global community for women to gather, share, and empower each other as a collective.

TheeSisterNet@gmail.com

don't forget to breathe.

READY

"Where there is ruin, there is hope for treasure." -Rumi

The words were inscribed on her heart. She'd tattooed them there on a nondescript night, where nothing particularly exciting had marked the hours, so she was never able to recall the date.

But there was a vibration between the words...that hummed like a lullaby's melody - born to soothe, to comfort. She knew for certain that life's bumps would call for them.

So she saved them on her heart, where they sometimes drifted apart, and sometimes came together in new pairings...never wandering too far from the contemporaneous beat of her center.

And when her world came tumbling down, there they were, pirates after booty.

REFLECTION FIVE

Recently, I learned a new word - melomaniac. A melomaniac is a person with an excessive or abnormal fondness for music. When I learned that one's affinity toward music could be considered *excessive*, I also knew the word accurately described my relationship to the art form. Music is such a transformative craft. It connects me to people, places and things (all the nouns) in profound ways. Frequently, Rumi's words conjure the same response from me.

Complete a quick mental scan of your life experiences. Search for events that stand out for evoking a deeply rooted sense of connection. Capture those memories on the following pages. Consider how often you revisit these memories.

don't forget to breathe.

MY VOICE

Sit up straight.
Cross at the ankles.
Don't speak unless spoken to.
Is that it?

FAMILY

Abstain.
Submit.
In Jesus' name.
Is that it?

CHURCH

Less passion.
Too much emotion.
"We think John should lead this time."
Is that it?

CORPORATE

Be a lady.
Don't be prude.
Respect yourself.
Is that it?

SOCIETY

Crowded.
Confused.
Unsure.
That's it.

My voice

REFLECTION SIX

I once watched a film where the male character rejected the female character's description of getting to know him as "peeling back the layers of an onion". In rebuttal, he asserted that learning more about him was instead like peeling back the layers of an artichoke. He explained that the inside of an onion is just more onion, whereas at the center of an artichoke is a heart.

That scene stuck with me as a phenomenal example of self-awareness. More specifically, the male character's understanding of how he wanted to be defined and his having the courage to share his truth with someone with whom he hoped to grow closer.

If you have had such a moment of self-awareness and agency, take some time to reflect and revere your willingness to have and maintain a boundary.

If you have not had such an experience, take some time to imagine how you would like to show up in moments when you feel misrepresented by another person's definition of you.

don't forget to breathe.

YOU DESERVE

Can't completely wrap my mind around
how to let the words penetrate my consciousness.

In a way that feels
accepted
or
even considered.

How do others do it?

Do they do it;

let the words in,
in a meaningful way?

In a way that allows the words -
the essence of them,
the nutrients of them -

to settle in,
and grow,
and become,

a living breathing part of their "self" -
of who they know themselves to be,
of how they feel about themselves.

Some people radiate.
Some people glow.
Some people vibrate.

Are those the manifestations -
the harvests,
the personifications

of "you deserve"?

Do they know -
do they actively feel it in their cells,
and attached to their breath?

Is it evident in their way of being,
of receiving the world?

Is it just me?
Inept.

Are there more like me?
How do I find them?
Why haven't I found them?

Am I asking the wrong questions?

REFLECTION SEVEN

Curiosity is my jam! So is self-doubt. The two together sometimes run me ragged from the cyclical way they serve each other in my mind, fueling thoughts of catastrophe. But occasionally, the combination causes me to mirror another person in a way that leads to the cycle being broken. When I hear the words of self-doubt or catastrophizing mirrored back to me, it becomes easier to hear how counterproductive they are.

Think back to a time when behaviors or words you often perform or speak allowed you to have a reformative interaction, interrupting a habitual action or negative self-talk.

don't forget to breathe.

STILL

Bright lights flashing.

I am in bloom -
a bouquet of intrepid flowers.

Floating through time.

Where form is in the hands of the formed,
and my double consciousness is reconciled.
I told myself I was fine.

Everything was foreign;
anything was possible.

And love
was the only thing still certain.

REFLECTION EIGHT

One day, I used my weekly poetry class at Elizabeth's Bookshop & Writing Centre** as an excuse to explore outer space. I surrendered my mind to my curiosity. I did not try to push limits because I noticed that in surrendering, I forfeited all concepts of them.

I took on many forms with ease but held on to the light from Genesis 1:3 - the light that God ensured came before us, that made a way for us. I saw it in many forms, and it was surrounded by, or maybe made of, love every time.

Close your eyes. Let go of as many thoughts as your conscious mind will allow. Lose awareness of your earthly weight and ego. Take deep, intentional breaths in and long emptying breaths out. Once all you can hear is your breath, take a mental trip. There are no rules and no limits. Document where you permit yourself to go.

Elizabeth's Bookshop & Writing Centre: A Black-owned bookstore and literacy center that highlights, promotes, and honors the work of writers of color, LGBTQ+, disabled and other marginalized authors.
www.ElizabethsOfAkronShop.com

don't forget to breathe.

DISNEY: THE MINORITY REPORT

I have romanticized love for so long,
I don't know if I can get past its pain to realize its potential?

Whether I will forever fall victim to grandeur ideas of its fantasy,
and miss its fullness?

If it will ever be unconditional enough to weather the storms
of my insecurities?

I often wonder if it is made for me -
in this space, in this time?

Or

If it is my plight in this realm, to make do with the understanding that
there will be enough love in the next to overwhelm my soul?

REFLECTION NINE

The lies I tell myself can be suffocating. The lies I tell myself can also be distracting. The lies I tell myself are **always** an illusion. The original chameleons, lies can shapeshift however needed to maintain the illusion. It is important to remember that lies work only as hard as they have to for deception.

I have adopted the definition of 'lie' shared by Tina Lifford - Founder of The Inner Fitness Project - in - *"The Little Book of Big Lies" - any experience or event that leaves us feeling worthless, not good enough, afraid of discovering or being ourselves, or disconnected from our innate value; a false impression.* My poem *Disney: A Minority Report* is centered around the idea that this life does not hold love (or enough love) for me. That is an excellent example of a lie I told myself. The truth is, there is love all around me, and the more I grow and learn, the more I see it.

In this reflection, work to see the lies you have told yourself/ believed about yourself over the last day or week. Use this space to release as many lies as time and memory afford you.

***The Inner Fitness Project:** A wellbeing initiative that teaches reliable "inner" practices for navigating your past, present, and future.
www.TheInnerFitnessProject.com

don't forget to breathe.

DON'T FORGET TO BREATHE.

I was so sure that:
good and bad were finite
feelings were truth
love would never fade
I would never heal
I had more control
being responsible would make me worthy
if I didn't want to, I wouldn't
I would crumble under pressure
fear was my limit
that "one thing" was unforgivable
I would die young...

I could live off of grapes, forever.

REFLECTION TEN

The one thing about my imagination is that it is either busy expanding or limiting me. Never both things at once. When I find myself caught up in fairytale thinking or a spiral of catastrophizing, I take a moment to ask myself, "What did you do last time?"

For me, that question is grounding. It reminds me that this is not the first time I have experienced these feelings or these thoughts. And most importantly, after experiencing the thoughts or feelings, I am still here.

Deep inhale. Deep exhale. Repeat as many times as needed to bring you to the present moment. Recount the last time you felt desperate, unraveled, or uncertain. Remember how your body felt through each phase of desperation, unraveling, or uncertainty. Now, try to remember as many instances as possible where your body responded this way.

don't forget to breathe.

MORE

Bigger than words.
Bigger than worlds.

We were an experience.
Everyone could feel it.
Everyone loved it. (the feeling)

But we couldn't afford to hold on.

Not if we were going to grow.
Not if we were going to be, MORE.

Together, we were something.
What a beautiful moment.
What a magical ride.

Oooooohhhh what a feeling.

Now we are written in the stars,
for generations to look up,

and adore
and never settle
and never forget who they are to become.

REFLECTION ELEVEN

I learned these three things through experience: It's essential to set boundaries; some people will coexist with me only for a season; and temporary satisfaction does not typically outweigh the opportunity for growth that comes from doing the more challenging thing. None of those experiences were easy. All of the experiences allowed me to mature or solidify my maturity.

What I appreciate most about my current stage of emotional maturity is that I do not always need the benefit of hindsight to know that even the things that hurt me can later be used in the testimony of a "greater good".

Which life lesson(s) contributed to you building or honing your favorite characteristics about yourself and your values?

don't forget to breathe.

REMEMBER
BY EBANEE BOND

Written December 16, 2022 at 10:53pm

When life has been a terror for years,
years later
you must remember what you loved —
how you loved cooking,
giving thoughtful gifts,
birds chirping,
and new Beyonce.

It's as if you loved life and
life loved you.
It's as if you lived life and
life lived through you.

Love dwelled —
remember?

Life has been hard on you.
It hasn't been jovial.
It hasn't been inspired.

Please,
glimpse into!

Remember!
When you were…

Love

www.EbaNeeBond.com

REFLECTION TWELVE
BY EBANEE BOND

Until roughly my early twenties, I had such a strong sense of self and zeal for life. About a decade later, I was at an event and someone asked me, 'What brings you joy?' At that moment, I realized I didn't know. How could I possibly be living a life without joy?

Between my early twenties and early thirties, my brain had been so altered by trauma that imminent danger shrouded my view. It seems the pain came one day and just decided to linger, forever coloring my world with gloom. I wrote this poem because I wanted to rewire my brain to be a receptor to a good life by triggering it with past splendid moments and giving it hope that joy is still possible. I wanted to take more control of painting the world on the screens of my mind.

I read somewhere that the experiences we enjoyed doing don't stop being enjoyable; we just stop doing them. What are some experiences from different periods of your life, including your childhood, that brought you satisfaction or joy to do them?

don't forget to breathe.

AFTERWORD
By Vanessa Flowers

Have you heard the saying – when a flower doesn't bloom, you fix the environment in which it grows, not the flower? I believe growth involves awareness and realizing our role in the process. It also calls for leaving environments not meant for us. Growing is hard and can feel so painful at times because we're bending in new ways. But it is also a beautiful process to experience our evolution and become aware of our potential. When we leave unhealthy environments and relationships, we're able to relieve tension and realize we're not alone in our struggles. And when we become aware of the role we play in our own suffering, we can humble ourselves to life's unpredictable circumstances.

I love *don't forget to breathe*. because it's a reminder to breathe through even our most trying challenges. We have to pause and become aware of what's not worth our energy and invite what is. When we breathe, we buy ourselves time to be present, to figure out our wants and needs. Each poem in the book is written with such rawness that you can tell Ceyanna is speaking from experience, and with each reflection you're reminded to pause and think about the ways we speak to ourselves. Is it coming from a place of love? Grace? Peace? Breathe easy and know that life will bless you with everything you want and more if you believe.

I met Ceyanna many years ago when we worked alongside one another. The thing I admire about her most was her willingness to take a breath, find calmness within herself and learn how to do new challenging things. She was open to admitting what she didn't know and excited to learn something new. Everyone admired her ability to keep cool, which stems not only from her character but also from practice and experience. Trust and know that everything she's writing in this book is full of wisdom and strength. Know that she's coming from a place of love and wanting you to live your most authentic life! Healing is hard, and you'll feel like you're falling apart at times, but that's okay. As my Aunt Toni always says, "Embrace every part of your journey!"

I pray you learn to give yourself grace through it all because you are so worthy.